Hotel Fitness
Workouts for the Road Warrior

John Stefansson

CONTENTS

INJURY DISCLAIMER

Before beginning any exercise regimen, consult your doctor. The author and publisher of Hotel Fitness disclaim any liability resulting from performing any of the activities contained in this book.

HOW TO USE THIS BOOK

This book goes over a wide range of topics on hotel fitness, from nutrition to the specific exercises to whole routines. I recommend you read the book in its entirety, from start to finish. I also recommend you actually do the exercises once you read about them. Then I recommend you translate this book line-by-line to Mandarin. Or not. It's just a recommendation.

WHO AM I AND WHY ARE YOU LISTENING TO ME?

Be honest with yourself. When was the last time you got a great workout at a hotel? If you are like most people, probably never. Ok, definitely never. Fun fact, up until I came up with this routine, I didn't either. I had never even sweated at a hotel. Ok that's a lie. The air conditioning in my room broke one time. Besides that though, not a bead.

When at home, I went to the gym regularly. The squat rack was my home away from home. So why did I not do anything when I was at a hotel? Excuses. Excuses such as:

"There is no time"
"They don't have my equipment"
"I can't get a good workout anyway"

Plus, who can resist the allure of boozing and schmoozing while you're on vacation? It was a matter of fact: when you went away, it was time to play. Thus a series of events were set in motion:

- You arrive at a hotel for vacation or some sort of business event
- You go for drinks later either with the client or your pals
- Everyone orders a beer and other calorie heavy food and drink
- You finish late at night and don't get a lot of shut eye
- You wake up the next morning feeling awful for what you have eaten
- Repeat

For someone who had been trying to get in shape, it seemed like a vicious cycle. I, like many people, wanted a way to burn off those calories but found the gym at the hotel lackluster. Because I found it lackluster I figured it wasn't worth going to the gym since I wouldn't get a good workout. This circular logic essentially trapped me. What I needed was a kick to get out of my current state. One time I went on an extended stay to Florida where many of my friends were stationed at the time. I was starting to form a beer gut, destroying all progress I had made that year at the gym. As any middle-aged man can tell you, a beer gut makes you look fantastic. Time for a change.

The first step to solving any problem is to identify it. Problem: the gyms at a hotel suck. Solution: Buy every hotel I go to and change the gym to make it not suck. Next problem: I don't have that much money. Solution: Become Bill Gates. So far so good. Except not really. I needed a more realistic plan.

The other way was to adapt my workouts on the road to make do with what I had. Often that was nothing more than a table, chair and some dumbbells. So I looked high and low for exercises that I could use or modify slightly so that I could still get a good workout while at a hotel. The military, body weight workout sites and prison gym routines all proved to be useful resources. I compiled them all and applied the various restrictions usually placed on hotel workouts i.e. equipment available, limited time, etc.

I reduced all the equipment needed to the following:

- Table
- Chair
- Towel

- Treadmill (optional)
- Jump Rope (For those that want to plan ahead)

One can bring a jump rope in a small bag if they wish to experience the full workout. Everything else is available at essentially any destination.

Next trip I was ready. The workouts were designed to take no more than an hour and a half. Depending on my schedule, I either woke up early or went right after the day's activities to get my fitness on. They were grueling and challenging exercises, not just substitutes to pass the time. At dinner, I drank water. If the occasion really called for alcohol, I'd get bourbon (less calories). Lo and behold, I started to lose weight. In fact, I got in great shape.

I got addicted to these body weight exercises. Even when I wasn't traveling I continually did more push-ups, more wall-sits, more everything with the body. I cut my gym membership. After all who wants to wait for all the weights to free up when I can do my work out essentially anywhere? The progress snowballed and I found myself competing in mud runs, 5k's and other forms of competitions. Life itself became easier. People inherently respect you more when you are in shape. It's the raw truth. Plus you feel good about yourself, because no else around you can belt out as many push-ups as you.

So who am I? I am your average Joe who wanted a change and wouldn't let my work stand in the way. I want to share it with you because losing weight is a worthy challenge that we all face at one point in our lives.

And if you don't travel? I got news for you. Body weight exercises work for everyone. They also don't cost money, unlike a gym membership. Even if you aren't ready to cut the cord on your membership yet, having a backup plan that can work essentially anywhere is invaluable.

Whatever reason you have for picking up this book, realize that I can only give you the tools to achieve. It is up to you to follow through, to be dedicated to change. Everyone wants to be in shape. So why aren't they? Because when the pain starts, when you have to decide between working out and watching TV they choose the easy path. Nothing in this world comes to you without hard work except your momma's love. Plan. Execute. Achieve. These three words will guide you on your journey. Learn to put all you have. The Spartan warriors believed that all were born equal and thus only those trained in the most severe school would win in battle. Make your school the most severe.

NUTRITION AND SLEEP

Did you know sleep is one of the key ingredients to recovery? Without it you'll never be able to achieve your fitness goals. You will, however, become a zombie. I hear they are all the rage now in Hollywood. Make sure to get a good agent. But seriously, sleep and nutrition are things that are in short supply while traveling. Often meetings run late, much caffeine is consumed and sleep is often considered a luxury. If you find yourself not being able to exercise daily I recommend that you consider a bi-daily routine. That is, workout one day and sleep well (a good 7-9 hours) on the next. This insures you won't turn into a complete zombie.

Nutrition is a little trickier. You can try a multitude of things: multi-vitamins, skipping the soda, etc. To be honest you are just trying to minimize damage. Eat a lot of protein, try to stay away from heavy carb food as there is no way you can burn off that much energy given your time constraints.

Despite this, there are actually some things that almost every hotel has that can help you achieve success. I have compiled a collection of things that almost every hotel has that will help you with your goal. Go to:

http://hotelfitnessbook.com

To download the free PDF.

However, in the end all one has to do is eat smart and your body will thank you.

JOHN STEFANSSON

THE EXERCISES

Push-Ups

Push-ups (or press-ups) are the quintessential bodyweight exercise. A classic among the military for punishment, it will become one of your cornerstones when exercising on the go. The standard push-up is the common one. Everyone knows it. However, if that were the only push-up game around the exercise would become easy. Fortunately, the human mind is great at coming up with new ways to inflict pain on itself and there are many variations.

Normal

These are the bread and butter of your to-go workout routine. Get on your stomach and put your palms slightly wider than shoulder width apart on the ground. Now push. There should only be four points of contact on the ground. Two of them are your hands, the other are either your toes or your knees, depending on your level.

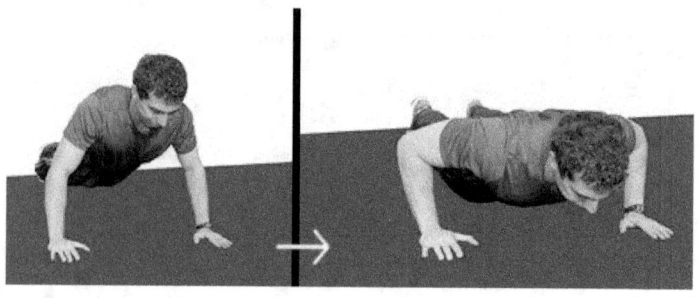

You should do these with gusto, it only gets better from here. I want you to practically hear the drill sergeant yell at you while you try and belt these out.

Wide

A slight variation on the normal push-up, the instructions are virtually identical with the exception that you should place your palms farther out.

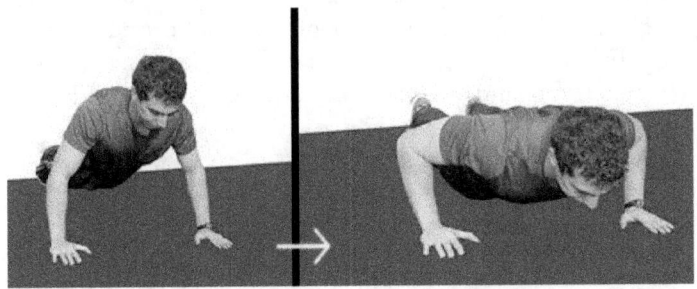

Remember that the further the arms go the less range of motion you have but the better the workout is. Find a balance.

Diamond

An athlete-maker. Not only do these work the biggest part of your arm (triceps) they keep you honest as to how strong you really are. Start on your stomach and put your hands together such that your index finger and thumbs are touching. You should get a roughly diamond outline from your fingers. Place the center of the diamond right under your sternum and push. Make sure to fully extend your arms. Do it right or don't do it at all.

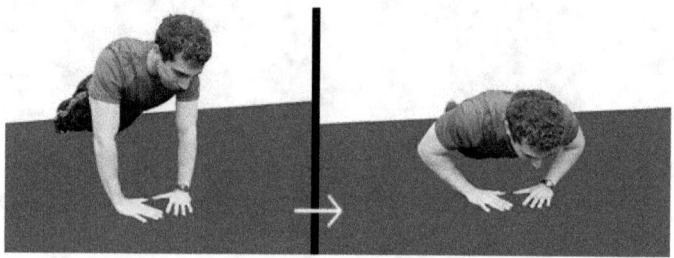

For a more advanced version, do these on a laminated floor (or something that gets slippery when wet). Why? When your hands start to sweat, the traction your hands had disappears and you have to use even more muscle to stabilize them.

Dive Bomber

Also known as the "I look like I am licking the floor" push-up. Congrats, everyone thinks you are crazy because you look ridiculous doing these. Fortunately, they are worth every odd stare that comes your way.

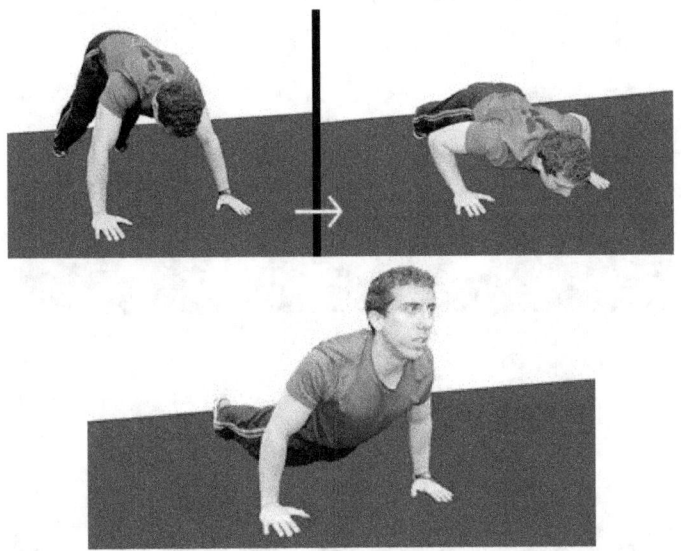

Start with your hands and toes on the floor shoulder width apart with your bum in the air. Now I want you to think that you are going to take a big lick of that germ-infested floor. Move your head in that way (without licking the floor since you want to remain healthy) and eventually arch your back without touching the floor. Pictures do it more justice than words.

This is an exercise that feels easy when done wrong. You'll know when you are doing them right.

Rotation

Do a standard push-up, but when you have extended your arms rotate to a side and reach up to the sky like you need help from the heavens. Then realize that you actually like the burn. Rotate back and do another pushup. Repeat and make sure to alternate sides of rotation.

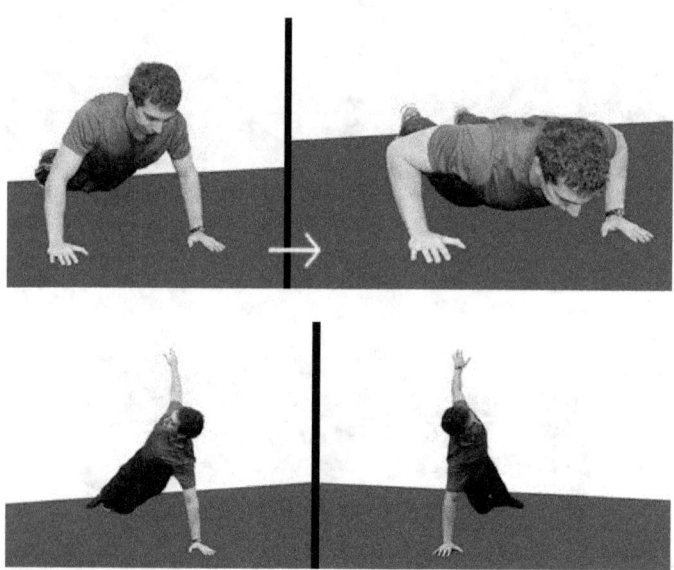

Goblet Squat

Place your feet slightly wider than shoulder width apart and make sure the toes point slightly outwards. Now squat down trying to make the back of your calves slightly touch the back of your thighs. Wait there for a couple seconds and come back up. Too easy? Grab something that is small and heavy. If you are lucky enough to be in a hotel with dumbbells or medicine balls, use them. Put the weight near your chest while you do them.

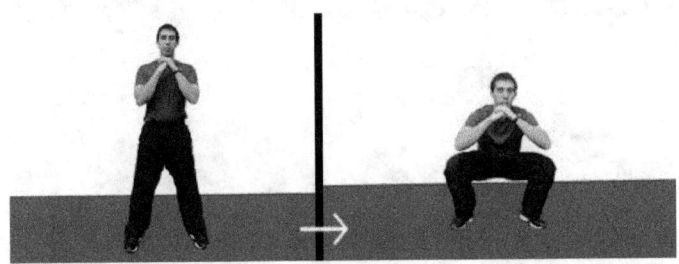

Burpees

These just suck. The only thing that sucks more is doing more of them.

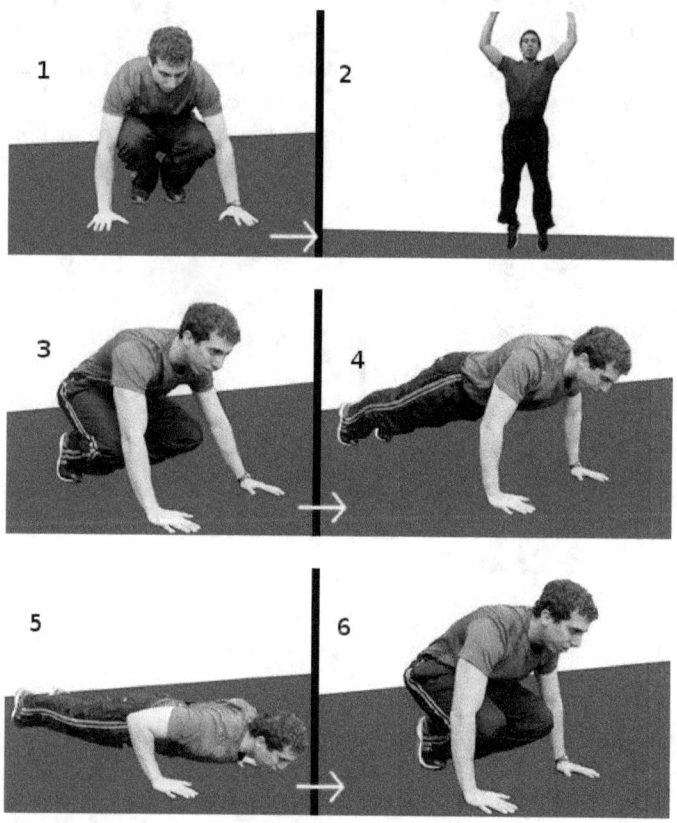

Start in a squatted position and jump up in the air, making sure that your feet leave the ground. Land in the same position. Then kick your feet out behind you and do a pushup. Jump back into the initial position. Repeat.

Lunges

Stand with your legs together. Take one large step forward so that even Neil Armstrong knows you mean business. Bend your knees so that your non-forward leg almost touches the ground. If it touches you lose.

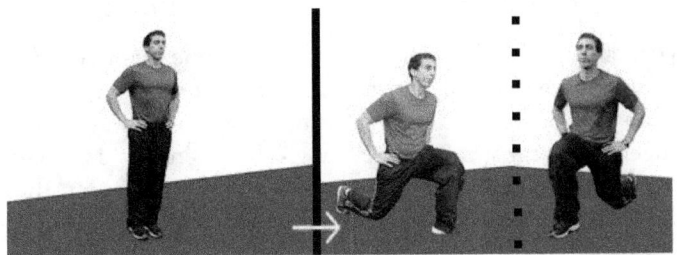

Make sure to keep your back straight and if you want some more pain carry some weights in each hand.

Abs

Question time. Let's say you have an 880 horsepower V8 engine, top-of-the-line tires and a space-age carbon fiber chassis. How fast will it go without a transmission system? Go ahead, I'll wait.

Back already? Of course you are. Anyone with a brain knows that without a transmission, it does not matter how much raw power you have, it cannot be transferred to the wheels and thus move the car. Why then do so many people ignore their abs? Your abs are the transmission that allow you to transfer power from your legs to your upper body and vice-versa. If you neglect your transmission you are going to regret it.

Sit-Ups

The arch-nemesis of the beer gut. Annihilate those persistent empty calories and destroy your lower back at the same time! Seriously though, even though the sit-up is a classic, there are many modern twists that improve on it. I include it for nostalgia purposes.

Sit on your bum and make it so that your legs form a pyramid outline. Cross your arms across your chest like a mummy and bring your chin to your knees. Go back down and repeat.

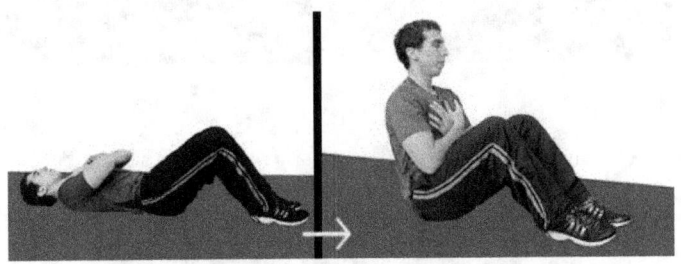

Bicycle Ab Workout

A more elegant workout for a more civilized age. Better than your standard sit-up and it does not kill your lower back, this should be the go-to work out for anything ab related.

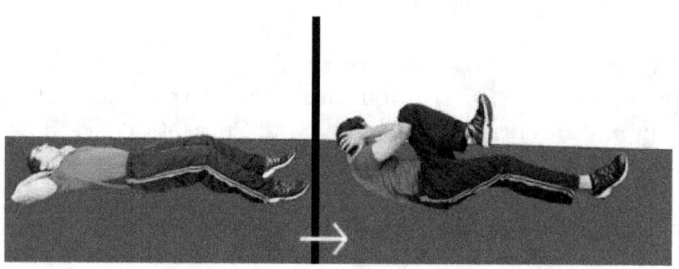

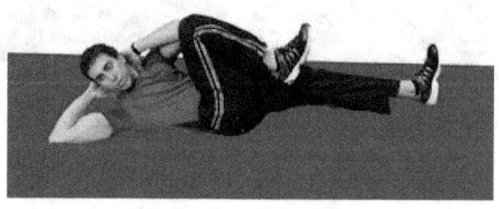

Start on your back and put both hands behind your head. Lift your legs off the ground and bring one of your knees up. Touch it with the opposite side elbow. Go back to your original position and repeat while making sure to alternate sides. One repetition is counted when you have returned to the original leg/elbow combo.

Reverse Sit-up

If you just love your damn sit-ups then at least do the reverse sit-up. If you have a bench then lay down on it and grab the edge near your head with your hands. If not, lay down on the ground and keep your hands palm down near your sides. Keep your feet together and bring your knees to your head. Then kick up your legs towards the ceiling. Reverse the procedure to get back to the starting position.

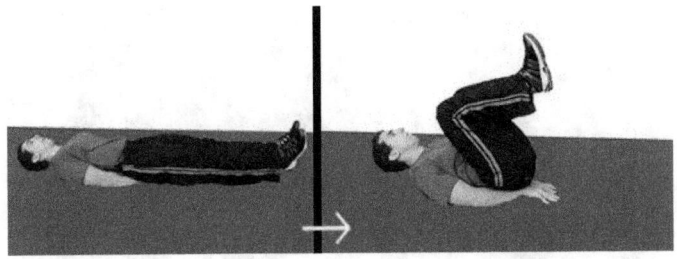

Plank

One of the better static exercises and a rumored favorite of famous martial artist Bruce Lee. Get on your stomach and put your forearms underneath you. You should have four points of contact, your toes and your forearms. Keep your back straight, no bums in the air or floor draggers.

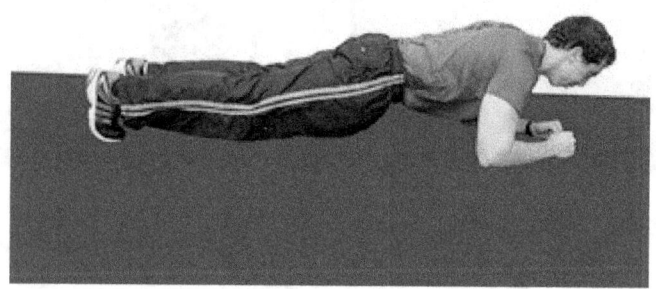

Side Plank

Instead of a normal plank, rotate to one side and utilize your sides to maintain this static position.

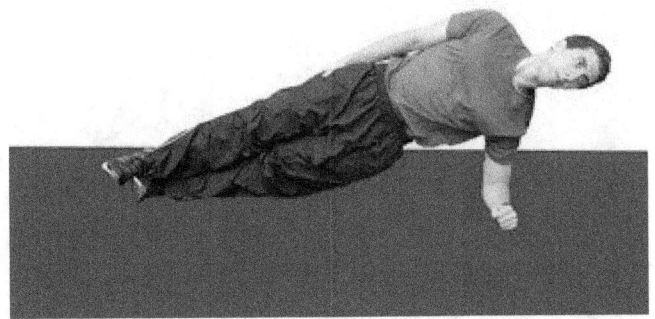

Single Leg Plank

Similar to a normal plank but you have three points of contact instead of four: two forearms and one toe

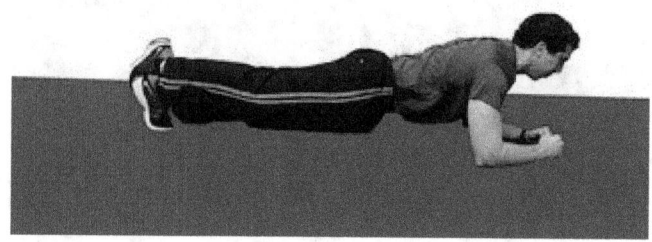

Dips

Your triceps make up roughly 2/3 of your arm. Forget curls, forge your arms with dips. Sit down on the edge of a chair. Put your palms on the edge of the chair with your fingers pointing to your legs. Push yourself slightly forward with your arms and dip down with your arms until they form a 90 degree angle. Remember, you want your arms to form a corner, not an acute angle.

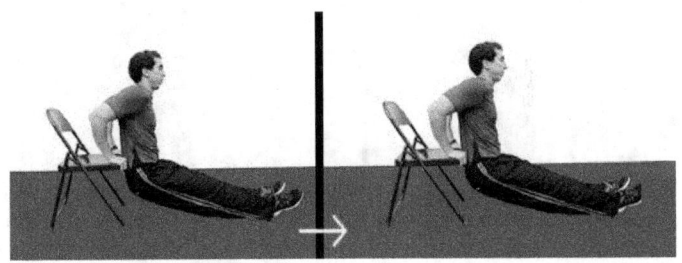

Jumping Jacks

Also known as the star jump, this is a great exercise to warmup and get your heart pumping. Start by standing up straight with your arms to your sides. Slightly jump then simultaneously separate your legs and move your arms above your head. If you are worried about rotator cuff issues, you can do so called "half-jacks" which means that you move your arms halfway up instead of all the way.

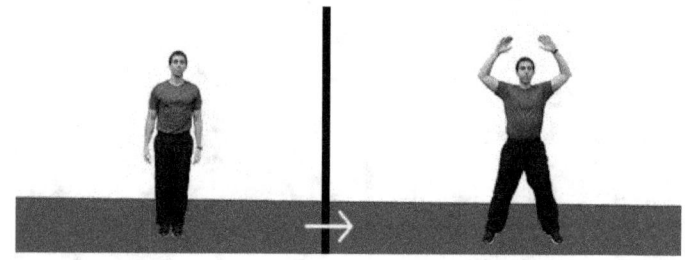

Jump Rope

This exercise only applies if your location of travel has a small rope or if you had the foresight to bring a rope. Although jumping rope is good for your body, it really trains your central nervous system. Use it for warm up and you'll feel sharper as you lift.

Although there are many variations, the one I feel works best is the standard rope skip with hand crossing. Simply jump the rope at an ever increasing rate until you feel you have reached your limit. Hold this rate and every once in a while cross your hands across your body and jump through the corresponding loop. Resume your initial position and continue at the rate you were going at.

Step Ups

Take a chair and put its back against the wall. Now step on the chair and step down. BOOM! Mission accomplished. It's so easy I doubt you even needed this explanation. Want to make it harder? Carry some weight while you do it.

Wall Sit

Hate sitting in chairs? Man, have I got the workout for you. Lean against the wall. Now slide down until your thighs are parallel to the ground. Sit there with your legs burning and contemplate how you actually like sitting in chairs.

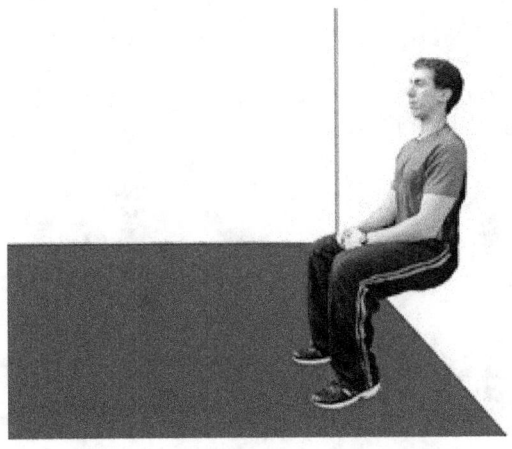

Dynamic Chest Extension

An exercise that I use to decompress after a heavy workout. It makes you use your muscles to hold a static position which seems to really help with removing the burn that come from other workouts. Stand up straight with a chair held by your hands near your chest. Extend your arms so that they are as straight as possible without locking them. Hold the chair there for the specified time and then return the chair. If you want to make it more challenging, put more weight on the seat of the chair.

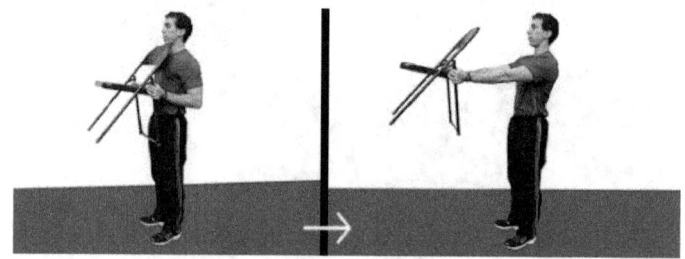

Arm Static Pull

Another workout I use to decompress. Take a medium sized towel and grab it with both hands palm down. Make sure your hands are slightly less than shoulder width apart. Now bring your arms up to neck level and try to pull the towel apart. Hold this static position for as long as it is specified.

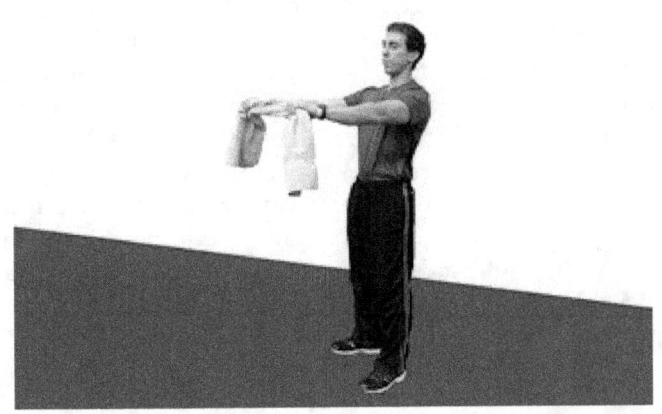

Inverted Bodyweight Row

Inverted bodyweight rows are used here because most places you travel to do not have a pull-up bar. If they do, then substitute inverted bodyweight rows with pull-ups on a 1:1 ratio.

These babies are probably the best bodyweight exercise you can do besides pull-ups. However unlike pull-ups which require a pull-up bar, there are a variety of places that inverted rows can be done. Because you will be traveling, I find that the best place to do inverted rows is underneath a table. But in reality any bar that you can hang under will work. A popular alternative to the table is underneath the arms of a treadmill if your location has one.

To do an inverted row, lie on your back with your head directly under the edge of the table. Grab the edge of the table with your hands, palms facing your feet. Now pull yourselves up, sort of like a reverse push-up. Repeat as specified.

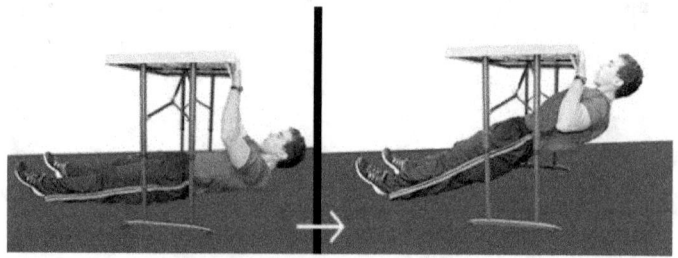

This exercise can be modified to work different parts of your body. Put your hands close together when grabbing the edge to work on your triceps. Spread your hands farther apart to work more on your back. Go to the other edge of the table and grab the edge with your palms facing your head. There are many analogous pull-up exercises that can be substituted if you do indeed have access to a pull-up bar.

WARMUP AND STRETCHING

General Overview

Did you know that the first shot fired out of barrel of a snipers gun is different than when he has "warmed" the barrel up? It is called a "cold bore" shot. Have you ever seen the starting lap of an F1 race? Wonder why they weave back and forth so fast? It is to warm up the tires so they can perform at the level they want.

"Warming up" is a fact of sports and life. Things just perform better once they get out of the "transient" state. This section outlines how to get the juices flowing and make sure you have everything you need to perform at your best.

Before you start your exercise and even before you warmup, a few people always ask me about "pre-workout" while on the road. For those of you who don't know, "pre-workout" is a supplement you take to get you ready and focused. Now unless you brought your pre-workout supplement with you, I would recommend taking a cup (or two) of coffee along with a banana as a make-shift substitute for pre-workout. The best part about this type of pre-workout is that many hotels/destinations of travel offer free coffee and fruit! Now onto the warmup.

The Warmup Routine

The point of the warmup is to get your heart pumping and to do that we need some intense exercises. The only two pieces of equipment you need are a treadmill and a jump rope. Both are optional, although if you are serious about fitness you should always pack a jump rope on your travels. Whether your destination has a treadmill or not is a crapshoot.

The warmup is the following:
- 7 minutes of treadmill at a medium-fast pace (If no treadmill is available do 50 burpees)
- 20 standard pushups as fast as possible
- 50 jumping jacks
- 2 minutes of jump rope (Optional)

After the warmup it is important to stretch. Also remember to stretch after completing the workout for the day as it is important to "reset" your muscles to a relaxed state after tightening them with the workout. Stretches after a workout should be held for thirty to sixty seconds each.

The following is a basic stretch routine, feel free to add stretches to it but do not skip any of the stretches listed here unless you have a replacement stretch. Even if you are not working a part of your body that day, you should stretch it to improve blood flow and thus make it stronger.

Neck Stretch

If you think you don't ever need to stretch your neck you are in for a big surprise. The neck muscles can tighten when you run and generally lock up when exerting effort using your traps. Also, try turning your head without your neck. Yup, impossible. So let's not let it get too stiff.

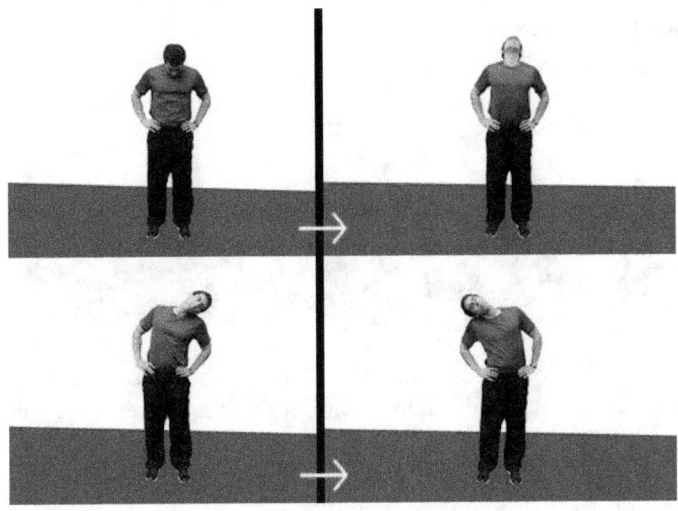

Luckily it is really easy to stretch your neck. Stand with your hands on your hips and start rocking your head back and forth, then side to side. Now roll your head around making sure to really get those muscles stretching. Do this routine a couple of times until you are satisfied.

Arm Stretches

Time to warm up the big guns. Nothing worse than having a cramp in your arm, so stretch them out so they can fire on all pistons. Start by crossing your right hand across your chest. Then wrap your left arm under and up to form a 90 degree angle. Now slightly pull with your left hand back and to your left to stretch your arm. Reverse the arm positions to stretch the other arm.

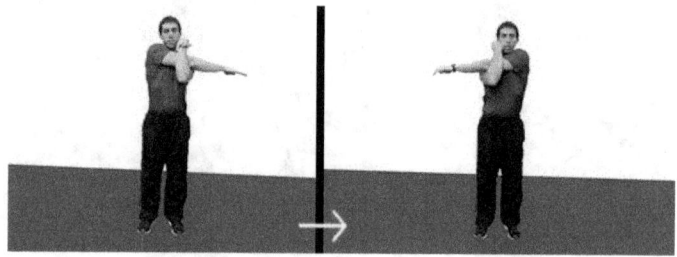

Now for another stretch. Take your right arm and reach for the sky. Now bend the arm so that your right hand touches your left shoulder muscle. Take your left hand and grab your right elbow and pull it to your left. Reverse arm positions to stretch the other arm.

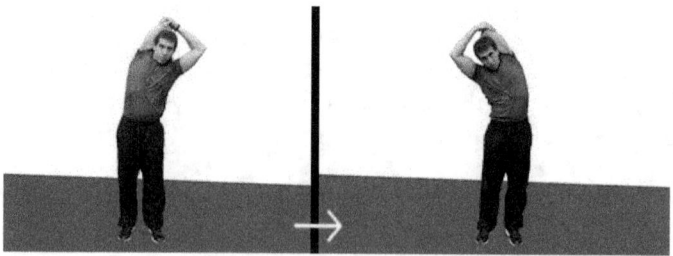

Stomach Stretch

Your core is your transmission system. You don't want to burn it out. There are a number of stomach stretches one can do, one of which is the "seal" stretch. Lie on your stomach, and push up with your arms while keeping your groin area on the ground. Try to arch your back and keep looking at that glorious ceiling. If this stretch seems too easy I recommend the other seal stretch where you join the US Navy SEALs and become an elite operator. After a couple of tours your stomach will be nice and flexible.

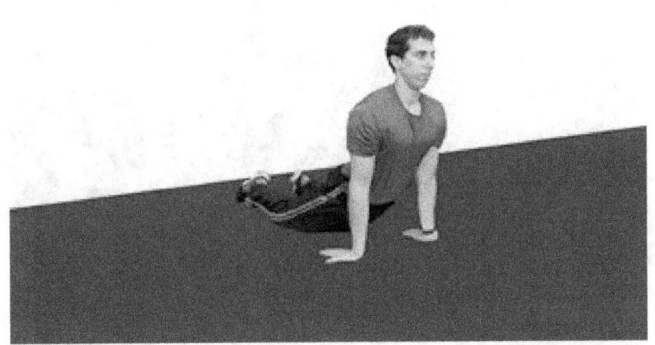

Groin Stretch

Colloquially known as the "butterfly" stretch, every student who has had physical education knows this stretch. Sit on the ground and put the soles of your feet together. Now bring those feet closer to your groin so your legs form a diamond. Grab at your ankles and bend forward while simultaneously breathing out. Try to stretch as far as possible and hold that position. Use your elbows to push down your knees to get a better stretch.

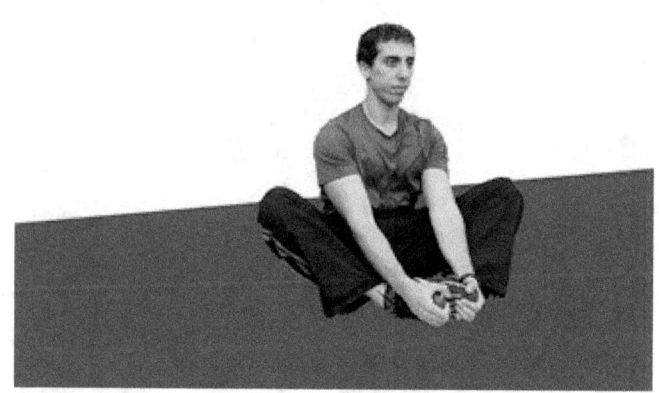

Calf Stretch

Stand facing a wall and bring one foot back so that it looks like you are trying to push said wall. Lean forward and keep that back heel stuck on that floor. If you don't feel the stretch, put your foot farther back and try again. Switch legs to stretch out both of your body movers.

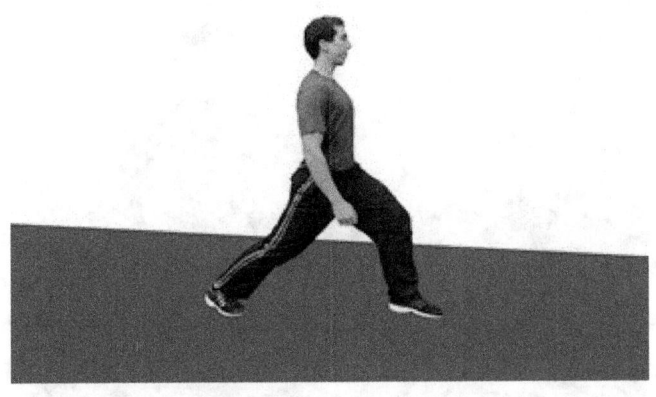

Ham String Stretch

Another muscle that has quite a few stretches for it. The one I use is perhaps the easiest. Simply sit on your bum and reach for your one of your feet, grabbing your toes. Place the sole of the foot that isn't being grabbed against the thigh of your engaged leg. Switch legs after completing one side.

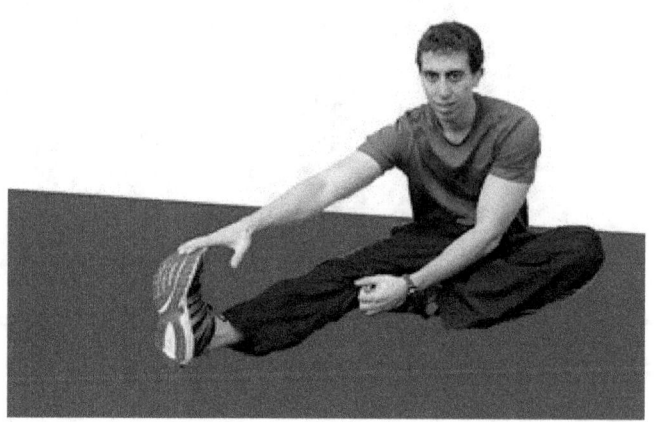

THE EXERCISES ROUTINES

General Overview

With the workouts defined, we can get to routines that can be done while traveling. Since one is not likely to stay at a location for an extended period of time, only three 1-week sample routines are shown here. These 1-week routines can be done in any order and you can feel free to create your own!

The theory behind each week is to alternate days of high intensity workouts with high-rep compound bodyweight exercises in order for your body to recover. If you decide to create your own schedule, follow this theory as much as possible in order to maximize your recovery.

To read the tables, it is important to understand the following:

- Make sure to start and end each day with a warm up as defined in the warm up section of this writing
- The syntax for each workout type
- What a set and a rep is

Before delving into the syntax, let us quickly review what a set and rep is. A set contains a number of reps. So for instance if I have to do five sets of four reps then for the first set I do four reps. I then rest and then begin set two, which again results in four reps. I continue this until I reach the end of set five. Why not just do twenty reps? Well some workouts might be hard enough that one cannot simply do twenty of them in a row. Plus this structuring allows one to take breaks at uniform intervals, which allows better measuring of progress.

Syntax for the Workouts

Due to the nature of bodyweight exercises, different set structures have been setup, including High Intensity Training (HIT) regimens. The types included in this book are Pyramids, HIT-type, Repeat-type and Regular. Feel free to modify them or add your own! The following subsections describe the general syntax of the workout and allows you to understand them. An example is also given with each general syntax.

Regular

Workout 1 - Number of Sets x Rep/Time Constant

Examples

Standard Pushups - 4x5
Wall Sit - 2x30 Seconds
Lunges - 1x30

When the workout instructs you to just do a regular exercise without any overbearing structure, it will look like it does above. The Rep/Time Constant specifies the number of reps or the time required for each set. For instance, a wall sit does not have a rep constant but a time constant. Conversely, pushups have a rep constant not a time constant.

For the regular example, we see that we must do the following: four sets of five reps of standard pushups, two thirty second reps of wall sits and one set of thirty lunges for each leg (meaning thirty with your left leg forward and thirty with your right leg forward). This results in a total of twenty pushups, one minute of wall sits and sixty lunges completed.

Pyramid

Pyramid (Level Start - Level End)
- Workout 1 x Multiplier
- Workout 2 x Multiplier

Example

Pyramid (1-5)
- Standard Pushups x 2
- Bicycle Ab workout x 3

This pyramid syntax would result in you starting with level one and maxing out with level five. At each level you are to do the workouts as listed from top to bottom with the number of reps being the current level multiplied by the workout multiplier. For this example, level one would result in you doing two standard pushups and three bicycles. Then you would progress to level two where you would do four standard pushups and six bicycles. This pattern would continue until you reached level five where you would do ten standard pushups and fifteen bicycles.

After you reach the "top" of the pyramid, you start at the top level and then work your way down to the starting level. So for this example, the levels done would go like:

1,2,3,4,5,5,4,3,2,1

This would result in a total of sixty standard pushups and ninety bicycles.

HIT-Type

HIT(Workout Length) x Repeat Constant
- Workout 1
- Workout 2
- Workout 3

Example

HIT(30)x2
- Standard Pushup
- Bicycle Ab Workout
- Inverted Bodyweight Row

The workout length is the number of seconds that you must do each workout. You must continually do each workout for the specified workout length. All HIT workouts involve a ten second rest between workouts. The repeat constant is the number of times you repeat each workout sequence.

In the HIT example, you would do the following:
1. Standard Pushups continually for 30 seconds
2. Rest 10 seconds
3. Bicycle ab workout continually for 30 seconds
4. Rest for 10 seconds
5. Inverted Bodyweight Rows continually for 30 seconds
6. Rest for 10 seconds
7. Repeat steps 1-6 a second time due to the repeat constant being two.

Repeat-Type

Repeat - Repeat Constant
- Workout 1 x Rep Number
- Workout 2 x Rep Number

Example

Repeat - 4 Times
- Standard Pushup x 5
- Plank x 15 Seconds
- Wide Pushup x 5

The repeat type of workout is simply you doing the listed exercises at their rep count in order. After completing all workouts, you rest for thirty seconds. If your repeat constant is higher than 1, you must repeat workout the specified number of times.

This example would result in one doing five standard pushups, a fifteen second plank and five wide pushups. Following a thirty second resting period, you would repeat this workout set three more times. This would result in twenty standard pushups, a full minute of planking and twenty wide pushups.

Using the Workout Routines

There are three workout routines shown below, separated based on current physical fitness levels into: novice, intermediate and advanced. How do you choose between the three? Generally speaking, if you cannot do a single pull-up or generally are not in shape, then go with the novice level. If you have been working out for a few years, go with intermediate. If you can squat and bench twice your body weight, or do marathon length obstacle courses, go advanced.

There is no shame in changing your level or only changing levels on certain days as you progress your workout. The point is to make sure that you are pushing yourself at an adequate level so that your level of fitness is improved, even while traveling.

Example of Using the Routines

You have been working out for about two years. During that time you can bench about your body weight and can do a fair number of pull-ups. You also have competed in some 5000 meter races without a lot of struggle. You decide that you will start with the intermediate workout table and adjust as necessary.

You fly out to your business hotel on Sunday and evaluate your room. The room itself has a table, a towel and a chair along with a bed. You check the fitness room and see two treadmills and a couple ten pound dumbbells. You also packed your trusty jump rope.

Monday roles around and you do your warmup and stretching as defined earlier in this writing. You try the intermediate "pyramid" workout and think it is too easy so you decide that next time there is a "pyramid" workout, you will do the advanced workout.

Tuesday you go in the gym and think because last workout was too easy you will go to the advanced High Intensity Training (HIT) workout. Unfortunately, your HIT training has been severely lacking and it takes too much out of you. You again modify your workout to be advanced "pyramid" sets with intermediate "HIT" sets.

This setup works well until Friday comes, when you have to catch a plane at midnight. You realize you don't have time to do the advanced pyramid set, so you settle for doing an easy pyramid set since something is better than nothing. Landing in your hometown, you realize that you have both travelled to a place that is out of the way while maintaining the fitness level you desired. You even now decide to incorporate HIT into your daily workout so you can do the advanced level of HIT next business trip.

Novice Workout

Monday - Week 1 - Novice
Pyramid (1-5)
- Inverted Bodyweight Row x 1
- Standard Pushup x 2
- Bicycle Abs x 2
- Dips x 2

Tuesday - Week 1 - Novice
HIT(15) x 1
- Jumping Jack
- Burpees
- Lunges
- Pushup and Rotation
- Front Plank
- Side Plank (Both sides)
- Reverse Sit-up
- Goblet Squat
- Wall Sit
- Step up

Wednesday - Week 1 - Novice
Pyramid (1-5)
- Standard Pushup x 1
- Wide Pushup x 1
- Diamond Pushup x 1
- Dive Bomber Pushup x 1

Pyramid (1-5)
- Bicycle Abs x 2
- Reverse Abs x 2
- Side Plank x 10 Seconds

Thursday - Week 1 - Novice
Burpees - 1x30
Lunges - 1x30
Goblet Squat - 1x30
Jumping Jacks - 1x80
Dynamic Chest Extension - 5x30 Seconds
Arm Static Pull - 5x30 Seconds

Friday - Week 1 - Novice
Pyramid (1-5)
- Inverted Bodyweight Row x 1
- Standard Pushup x 2
- Bicycle Abs x 2
- Dips x 2

Monday - Week 2 - Novice
Repeat 4 Times
- Standard Pushup x 5
- Bicycle Abs x 5
- Diamond Pushup x 5
- Plank x 15 Seconds
- Wide Pushup x 5
- Wall Sit x 15 Seconds

Tuesday - Week 2 - Novice
Pyramid (1-5)
- Inverted Bodyweight Row x 1
- Standard Pushup x 2
- Bicycle Abs x 2
- Dips x 2

Wednesday - Week 2 - Novice
HIT(15) x 1
- Jumping Jack
- Burpees, Lunges
- Pushup and Rotation
- Front Plank
- Side Plank (Both sides)
- Reverse Sit-up
- Goblet Squat
- Wall Sit
- Step up

Thursday - Week 2 - Novice
Pyramid (1-5)
- Inverted Bodyweight Row x 1
- Standard Pushup x 2
- Bicycle Abs x 2
- Dips x 2

Friday - Week 2 - Novice
Repeat 4 Times
- Standard Pushup x 5
- Bicycle Abs x 5
- Diamond Pushup x 5
- Plank x 15 Seconds
- Wide Pushup x 5
- Wall Sit x 15 Seconds

Monday - Week 3 - Novice
HIT(15) x 1
- Jumping Jack
- Burpees
- Lunges
- Pushup and Rotation
- Front Plank
- Side Plank (Both sides)
- Reverse Sit-up
- Goblet Squat
- Wall Sit
- Step up

Tuesday - Week 3 - Novice
Burpees - 1x30
Lunges - 1x30
Goblet Squat - 1x30
Jumping Jacks - 1x80
Dynamic Chest Extension - 5x30 Seconds
Arm Static Pull - 5x30 Seconds

Wednesday - Week 3 - Novice
Pyramid (1-5)
- Inverted Bodyweight Row x 1
- Standard Pushup x 2
- Bicycle Abs x 2
- Dips x 2

Thursday - Week 3 - Novice
Burpees - 1x30
Lunges - 1x30
Goblet Squat - 1x30
Jumping Jacks - 1x80
Dynamic Chest Extension - 5x30 Seconds
Arm Static Pull - 5x30 Seconds

Friday - Week 3 - Novice
HIT(15) x 1
- Jumping Jack
- Burpees
- Lunges
- Pushup and Rotation
- Front Plank
- Side Plank (Both sides)
- Reverse Sit-up
- Goblet Squat
- Wall Sit
- Step up

Intermediate Workout

Monday - Week 1 - Intermediate
Pyramid (1-7)
- Inverted Bodyweight Row x 1
- Standard Pushup x 2
- Bicycle Abs x 3
- Dips x 2

Tuesday - Week 1 - Intermediate
HIT(20) x 2
- Jumping Jack
- Burpees
- Lunges, Pushup and Rotation
- Front Plank
- Side Plank (Both sides)
- Reverse Sit-up
- Goblet Squat
- Wall Sit
- Step up

Wednesday - Week 1 - Intermediate
Pyramid (1-7)
- Standard Pushup x 2
- Wide Pushup x 2
- Diamond Pushup x 2
- Dive Bomber Pushup x 2

Pyramid (1-7)
- Bicycle Abs x 2
- Reverse Abs x 2
- Side Plank x 12 Seconds

Thursday - Week 1 - Intermediate
Burpees - 1x30
Lunges - 1x60
Goblet Squat - 1x60
Jumping Jacks - 1x120
Dynamic Chest Extension - 5x30 Seconds
Arm Static Pull - 5x30 Seconds

Friday - Week 1 - Intermediate
Pyramid (1-7)
- Inverted Bodyweight Row x 1
- Standard Pushup x 2
- Bicycle Abs x 3
- Dips x 2

Monday - Week 2 - Intermediate
Repeat 8 Times
- Standard Pushup x 5
- Bicycle Abs x 5
- Diamond Pushup x 5
- Plank x 15 Seconds
- Wide Pushup x 5
- Wall Sit x 15 Seconds

Tuesday - Week 2 - Intermediate
Pyramid (1-7)
- Inverted Bodyweight Row x 1
- Standard Pushup x 2
- Bicycle Abs x 3
- Dips x 2

Wednesday - Week 2 - Intermediate
HIT(20) x 2
- Jumping Jack
- Burpees
- Lunges
- Pushup and Rotation
- Front Plank
- Side Plank (Both sides)
- Reverse Sit-up
- Goblet Squat
- Wall Sit
- Step up

Thursday - Week 2 - Intermediate
Pyramid (1-7)
- Inverted Bodyweight Row x 1
- Standard Pushup x 2
- Bicycle Abs x 3
- Dips x 2

Friday - Week 2 - Intermediate
Repeat 8 Times
- Standard Pushup x 5
- Bicycle Abs x 5
- Diamond Pushup x 5
- Plank x 15 Seconds
- Wide Pushup x 5
- Wall Sit x 15 Seconds

Monday - Week 3 - Intermediate
HIT(20) x 2
- Jumping Jack
- Burpees, Lunges
- Pushup and Rotation
- Front Plank
- Side Plank (Both sides)
- Reverse Sit-up
- Goblet Squat
- Wall Sit
- Step up

Tuesday - Week 3 - Intermediate
Burpees - 1x30
Lunges - 1x60
Goblet Squat - 1x60
Jumping Jacks - 1x120
Dynamic Chest Extension - 5x30 Seconds
Arm Static Pull - 5x30 Seconds

Wednesday - Week 3 - Intermediate
Pyramid (1-7)
- Standard Pushup x 2
- Wide Pushup x 2
- Diamond Pushup x 2
- Dive Bomber Pushup x 2

Pyramid (1-7)
- Bicycle Abs x 2
- Reverse Abs x 2
- Side Plank (12 sec)

Thursday - Week 3 - Intermediate
Burpees - 1x30
Lunges - 1x60
Goblet Squat - 1x60
Jumping Jacks - 1x120
Dynamic Chest Extension - 5x30 Seconds
Arm Static Pull - 5x30 Seconds

Friday - Week 3 - Intermediate
HIT(20) x 2
- Jumping Jack
- Burpees, Lunges
- Pushup and Rotation
- Front Plank
- Side Plank (Both sides)
- Reverse Sit-up
- Goblet Squat
- Wall Sit
- Step up

Advanced Workout

Monday - Week 1 - Advanced
Pyramid (1-10)
- Inverted Bodyweight Row x 1
- Standard Pushup x 2
- Bicycle Abs x 3
- Dips x 2

Tuesday - Week 1 - Advanced
HIT(40) x 2
- Jumping Jack
- Burpees
- Lunges
- Pushup and Rotation
- Front Plank
- Side Plank (Both sides)
- Reverse Sit-up
- Goblet Squat
- Wall Sit
- Step up

Wednesday - Week 1 - Advanced
Pyramid (1-10)
- Standard Pushup x 2
- Wide Pushup x 2
- Diamond Pushup x 2
- Dive Bomber Pushup x 2

Pyramid (1-10)
- Bicycle Abs x 2
- Reverse Abs x 2
- Side Plank x 13 Seconds

Thursday - Week 1 - Advanced
Burpees - 1x90
Lunges - 1x90
Goblet Squat - 1x90
Jumping Jacks - 1x200
Dynamic Chest Extension - 5x30 Seconds
Arm Static Pull - 5x30 Seconds

Friday - Week 1 - Advanced
Pyramid (1-10)
- Inverted Bodyweight Row x 1
- Standard Pushup x 2
- Bicycle Abs x 3
- Dips x 2

Monday - Week 2 - Advanced
Repeat 8 Times
- Standard Pushup x 10
- Bicycle Abs x 10
- Diamond Pushup x 10
- Plank x 30 Seconds
- Wide Pushup x 10
- Wall Sit x 30 Seconds

Tuesday - Week 2 - Advanced
Pyramid (1-10)
- Inverted Bodyweight Row x 1
- Standard Pushup x 2
- Bicycle Abs x 3
- Dips x 2

Wednesday - Week 2 - Advanced
HIT(40) x 2
- Jumping Jack
- Burpees
- Lunges
- Pushup and Rotation
- Front Plank
- Side Plank (Both sides)
- Reverse Sit-up
- Goblet Squat
- Wall Sit
- Step up

Thursday - Week 2 - Advanced
Pyramid (1-10)
- Inverted Bodyweight Row x 1
- Standard Pushup x 2
- Bicycle Abs x 3
- Dips x 2

Friday - Week 2 - Advanced
Repeat 8 Times
- Standard Pushup x 10
- Bicycle Abs x
- Diamond Pushup x 10
- Plank x 30 Seconds
- Wide Pushup x 10
- Wall Sit x 30 Seconds

Monday - Week 3 - Advanced
HIT(40) x 2
- Jumping Jack
- Burpees
- Lunges
- Pushup and Rotation
- Front Plank
- Side Plank (Both sides)
- Reverse Sit-up
- Goblet Squat
- Wall Sit
- Step up

Tuesday - Week 3 - Advanced
Burpees - 1x90
Lunges - 1x90
Goblet Squat - 1x90
Jumping Jacks - 1x200
Dynamic Chest Extension - 5x30 Seconds
Arm Static Pull - 5x30 Seconds

Wednesday - Week 3 - Advanced
Pyramid (1-10)
- Inverted Bodyweight Row x 1
- Standard Pushup x 2
- Bicycle Abs x 3
- Dips x 2

Thursday - Week 3 - Advanced
Burpees - 1x90
Lunges - 1x90
Goblet Squat - 1x90
Jumping Jacks - 1x200
Dynamic Chest Extension - 5x30 Seconds
Arm Static Pull - 5x30 Seconds

Friday - Week 3 - Advanced

HIT(40) x 2
- Jumping Jack
- Burpees
- Lunges
- Pushup and Rotation
- Front Plank
- Side Plank (Both sides)
- Reverse Sit-up
- Goblet Squat
- Wall Sit
- Step up

WHERE TO GO FROM HERE

Congrats! You made it to the end. Except you didn't. There is no end to training, to improving, to becoming a better, more in-shape person. Even if you spend most of your time at a hotel. I hope with this book that I was able to impart at least some wisdom and inspire you to take action with your life. So how you do you continue on the path you started and reach even greater heights?

First (and I know I keep repeating this), get your **FREE** eBook on the top 5 nutritional things that hotels serve. Why do I keep saying this? Because 90% of getting in shape is your diet. That's right. Even if you exercise 24/7 you still are going to need to eat. And what you eat shapes what you look like and how well you recover. So do yourself a favor and pick up a complimentary copy.

http://www.hotelfitnessbook.com/

Second, you are going to need to surround yourself with likeminded people. With the internet, it doesn't matter whether you are in New York City or Japan, you can always connect with people who share your interests and motivate you to succeed.

Finally, you must personally change your own motivations so that you want exercise on the go. Now that you have read this book, you realize that you can get a good workout no matter where you are. Realizing that is half the battle. The other half is making sure you get up and do it. You can read about exercises until you are blue in the face but until you actually go and feel the burn you will never achieve your goals. The will to act. The tenacity to fail. The need to succeed. This is what separates the winners from the losers.

So what are you waiting for? Go get your fitness on.

"In practice we always base our preparations against an enemy on the assumption that his plans are good; indeed, it is right to rest our hopes not on a belief in his blunders, but on the soundness of our provisions. Nor ought we to believe that there is much difference between man and man, but to think that the superiority lies with him who is reared in the severest school."

- Thucydides